ISOMETRIC EXERCISES MADE SIMPLE

THE COMPLETE GUIDE AND HEALTH BENEFITS OF ISOMETRIC EXERCISES

ADREA HUFFMAN

Table of Contents

CHAPTER ONE

Isometric exercises

Exercising in an isometric position is called "isometric training

Doing isometric

Without moving the surrounding joints, Trusted Source exerts pressure on specific muscles. Isometric exercises can help to improve physical endurance and posture by strengthening and stabilizing the muscles through constant tension.

Isometric and isotonic muscle contractions are the two types of muscle contractions. Muscles undergo isotonic contractions when their length or length against resistance changes, but the tension does not. Isometric contractions occur when the muscle's length remains constant despite an increase in the muscle's stress.

Isotonic contractions are common in many strength-building exercises, such as concentric and eccentric movements. Muscles shorten when performed in a concentric manner, while lengthening when performed in an eccentric manner.

None of the muscles are shortened or lengthened during an isometric exercise. Isometric exercises don't change the shape or size of the muscles because the joints remain still. A typical isometric contraction can last anywhere from a few seconds to several minutes.

Isometric exercises can be done in a variety of ways, including by holding a specific position or by using weights. In order to increase metabolic stress on your muscles, hold the muscle contraction for a longer period of time. A good way to increase your strength and endurance is to do this.

Isometric exercises are easy to perform, don't require any equipment, and can easily be incorporated into a wide range of weightlifting exercises.

The Club Pilates instructor in New York, Femi Betiku, DPT, CSCS, explains that isometric exercises involve contracting a muscle or group of muscles and holding that position for the duration of an exercise. It's a departure from the typical strength training movement patterns: concentric (tension on a shortening muscle) or eccentric (tension on a longening muscle).

A plank is the simplest example of an isometric movement. While in the plank position, your entire core is tense and squeezed. It's an isometric contraction, and it's what you'd call a muscle contraction.

But many exercises incorporate all three movement patterns into their routines, such as the plank (which is an isometric exercise).

According to research "People forget that there is an isometric action in almost every exercise," research tells SELF in an email interview. In a squat, for example, you're in the eccentric phase when you lower the weight and your muscles lengthen. You're in the concentric phrase when your muscles contract as you return the weight. When you come to a halt and pause at the bottom, what happens in between? That's the isometric phase of the workout.

If you add a hold to a biceps curl, you can achieve the same results. The concentric portion is when you bend your elbow and curl the weight up. This is the part of the movement where you lower the weight by straightening your elbow and dropping it. This would be known as the "isometric" phase of the movement if you paused halfway through and held the 90-degree position of your arm.

Wall sits, calf raises, and hollow-body holds are all examples of isometric exercises. For those who prefer nonisometric exercises, holding them in a specific spot, such as just before you change direction, is an easy way to add an isometric component to your workout. As a bonus, it's a simple way to increase the difficulty of an exercise if you don't have the option of adding additional weight to the movement.)

CHAPTER TWO

Strength can be built through isometric exercises, but they do so in a different way than concentric and eccentric exercises. Nelson explains that with concentric and eccentric exercises, especially on the eccentric part, muscle fibers are broken down. The muscle tears that result from exercise will be repaired by the time you have given your body a chance to recover, and you will end up stronger than before as a result of those repairs.

Although Nelson claims that doing isometric exercises helps you build strength by strengthening your nervous system, this isn't entirely true. You're primarily training your nervous system to communicate with your muscles in a specific position and to activate the right muscles at the right time when you do isometric exercises.

While this isn't the most efficient way to build muscle, you can still use this method to build or maintain strength.

Even without alterations to muscle structure, says Nelson, "teaching the nervous system to get more muscle fibers to contract and coordinate" can lead to improved performance.

Muscular endurance, or the ability to hold a muscle contraction for a long period of time, is also a benefit of isometrics, according to Betiku.

This is why they're so effective at enhancing structural

steadiness. Doing a plank for long periods of time trains your entire core to activate and remain stable in the contracted position you're currently holding. The more you work your core, the better you'll be able to engage and stabilize your body during other movements like lunges or even running, which both call for a strong and engaged core.

Isometric exercises are common in many workout routines, as well as more dynamic ones.

Many muscle fibers can be activated at the same time with these exercises.

For example, squats require more practice to perform with proper form than other dynamic movements, such as push-ups.

• They are suitable for people who are unable to move as a result of an injury or a medical condition. As an example, a 2012 study found that people with osteoarthritis can benefit from isometric exercises.

Blood pressure can be lowered by incorporating isometric exercise training into your daily routine.

Muscle stability and the ability to hold weight for longer periods of time can be improved with these exercises, according to a study conducted in 2015.

To alleviate lower back, knee and neck pain, some studies have found that isometric exercises may be beneficial.

CHAPTER THREE

The dangers of isometric training

Compared to many dynamic movements, isometric exercises are less taxing on the major muscle groups. Isometric exercises, despite their potential for safety, can still result in injury or worsen an existing injury.

Poor form when performing isometric exercises can also result in injury. A plank performed incorrectly, for example, can lead to increased lower back tension and, as a result, injury.

If an isometric exercise causes a person to feel any pain or discomfort, they should immediately stop.

How can you incorporate isometric exercises into your workout?

Using isometrics frequently is the best way to get the most benefit out of them.

In order to maintain healthy muscles and joints, Betiku recommends performing isometrics every time you work out. When performing weighted concentric and eccentric movements, it's important to keep your major muscles strong and stable by working them isometrically. According to him, reducing your risk of injury can be as simple as maintaining a strong mind-muscle connection while also practicing stability and endurance exercises.

A biceps curl or a squat is an example of an exercise where

Betiku recommends using isometrics at the point in the movement where you feel the most vulnerable. If you're having trouble holding a position, slow down and take note of where you feel the most discomfort. As Fetiku points out, "if you can pinpoint that area in your exercise, that's your weak point."

Hold for 30 seconds after you've finished your set, then lower to the weak spot. By including an isometric component, you can improve your ability to complete the entire exercise by strengthening your muscles in that specific position.

As Betiku suggests, straight-up isometric exercises can also be used to complement the muscle groups that you're working on. As an example, do a short plank series at the beginning or end of your workout for upper-body and/or core training. In terms of fatiguing the muscles, Betiku recommends incorporating a few isometric exercises that complement the concentric and eccentric work you are already doing.

Adding an isometric variation to an exercise can help you master it if you're having trouble performing it correctly. You can improve your form and get a better sense of your intended range of motion by practicing isometrics, as recommended.

In the case of someone who is unable to squat [to depth], I will have them lower into a squat with proper form and then hold it so that they remember how the contraction feels and looks. Because they've developed that mind-muscle connection, their form tends to be better in subsequent repetitions."

Common ISOMETRIC EXERCISE INSTRUMENTS.

When used as part of a comprehensive training regimen, isometric exercise can take many forms. Deceleration and reversing direction are essential for people moving through their environment, and this is true whether they are sprinting on a soccer field or taking a sip of water. Isometric exercises can help maintain and strengthen postures and improve joint stability, but they are not the most effective method for developing force production .Core training makes heavy use of isometric exercises.

Core training aims to improve spinal stability, intervertebral stability, and lumbar stability, as well as peripheral joint mobility, by developing optimal levels of stability For neuromuscular efficiency and intervertebral stability, isometric core exercises focus primarily on the local core musculature.

During an isometric movement, a joint is held in place while the rest of the body moves in the opposite direction. Squatting is an example where movement has to stop at the bottom of the position before returning to the upright position. As a result, the individual's ability to maintain good posture and avoid compensatory movement is put to the test. No matter how good you are at sports, you will eventually reach a point where you can no longer maintain your balance in any given posture

Injuries, poor neuromuscular control, fatigue, and strength could all be contributing factors to these thresholds .An athlete's ability to keep their body in a stable position during critical moments can be improved by isometric exercises. This could be done by putting the body in a position and level of strain close to the conditions in which compensations would occur and then holding the position. External forces and time under tension should be constant and progressive, so that an individual's ability to maintain the same posture under similar conditions should improve.

Isometric exercises are also commonly used in physical rehabilitation to treat a variety of neuromuscular and musculoskeletal conditions, including acute and long-term pain (Kendall et al., 2005; Kisner & Colby, 2007).

Individuals who are unable to move can benefit from isometric exercises.

In spite of the fact that traditional exercise and resistance training may be more effective at building strength and improving physical performance, some people may be too unstable or experience pain when moving to take part in traditional exercise activities A path to more traditional exercises requiring more stability and a wider range of movements may be opened up through consistent application in a physical rehabilitation setting.

Isometric exercises and how to perform them are shown here.

Isometric exercises target various muscle groups and come in a variety of forms.

CHAPTER FOUR

Isometric exercises that are popular include:

A plank of wood.

The core muscles can be strengthened by performing plank exercises, according to a study published in 2016. In order to do a plank:

A press-up position is the starting point.

Bend your elbows until your forearms are parallel to the floor.

The forearms should be under the shoulders, and the core muscles should be tight.

Hold this position for 10 seconds at first and gradually increase the time you spend in this position.

Sit on the wall 2.

The wall sit is a simple exercise that targets the thighs' muscle endurance without putting undue stress on the lower back. There are several ways to do a wall sit.

Stand shoulder-width apart in front of a wall about two feet away.

Lie back on the floor with your back against the wall and slowly lower yourself into a seated position.

3. Maintain core tension while bending knees to a 90-degree angle, as if sitting on a chair.

As long as you can, keep your hands on the hips in this position.

3. The gluteal bridge

With this exercise, you'll work on your gluteal muscles, which sit behind your quadriceps. Bridge your glutes in this manner:

Lay on the back with the knees bent upward so that the feet are on the floor, and keep your back straight. Extend the arms and turn the palms toward the sky, pointing them upward.

2. Using the arms for support, engage the core muscles and lift

the hips off the ground until the torso is in a straight line.

Keep your core muscles engaged as you hold this position.

It's all over.

The upper body, in particular the shoulders, will benefit from a dead hang workout. To do this exercise, follow these instructions:

Pull-ups should be performed with hands shoulder-width apart on a pull-up bar.

2. Lift the feet off the ground and cross them so that the body is suspended in the air.

For as long as possible, hold this position.

In-and-out lunges

As with the traditional squat, this exercise builds leg strength and endurance through the repetition of the movement.

To do this exercise, follow these instructions:

Standing at least shoulder-width apart, put your hands on your hips.

Slowly lower yourself into a squat position by bending your knees and pushing your hips back.

The arms should be moved forward at the bottom of the movement to help with balance.

Hold this position for a few more seconds.

Summary

Isometric exercises are designed to put stress on muscles without affecting the joints around them. Muscle endurance can be improved by doing these exercises. Planks and glute bridges are two examples of isometric exercises.

A medical condition or injury may limit a person's ability to move freely, so these are ideal for those individuals.

Improved muscle performance can be achieved through the use of isometric exercises.

THE END